Today is sh*t

Chris Reinhardt

Copyright © 2019 Chris Reinhardt

All rights reserved.

ISBN: 9781092347891

Independently published

DEDICATION

To all of those who have seen me in these sh*t days, weeks and months and loved me through it, in spite of myself and regardless.

Thank you for sticking around.

CONTENTS

	Acknowledgments	i
1	Today is shit	3
2	I try. Don't I?	5
3	Manic and Sad. How?	7
4	I'm a machine	9
5	Today is weird	13
6	Really?! I'm not allowed 'cause you say so?!	15
7	It sucks being a girl sometimes	19
8	This is not a good chapter	21
9	Millionaire	23
10	The End… of this week	27

ACKNOWLEDGMENTS

As with everything in my life and just like a Hollywood Oscar's acceptance speech, I would like to thank my family. My family, in this particular context and for this particular string of words same may dare to call a book, is my husband and my children.
My husband for all of his love. And my children, not only or their love which is kind of non-optional, but as an apology for the way I am, for the way I love them and for the way they will have been taught to love: Unmeasurably and Unconditionally until it kind of hurts.

1 TODAY IS SHIT

Today is shit.
End of Chapter.

Chris Reinhardt

2 I TRY. DON'T I?

It definitely isn't lack o f trying. I try. I try to try even.

I try to smile and I succeed but most of the times only on the outside. I try to speak and end up opening my mouth and speaking for England indeed but I fear by the end I am not quite sure what I said or if it made sense, I remember feeling it did but I can't be sure.

I try to do stuff. I managed a bunch of stuff and suddenly I get a headache. A bad one. One that makes me dizzy, annoyed, disappointed that I was trying so hard and now this. I don't fight them anymore. I stop. I rest. I used to fight them and then be left in a near constant state of agony. Not anymore, it's not worth it I don't feel. I need to rest so I rest. I feel a failure for resting. How can I? Hoew tired can I be from a couple of loads of laundry and changing the bedsheets? How can I justify this to myself? And then If eel shit 'cause I feel shit. Everyone rests. What exactly is my problem? Am I that much of a Narcisissist that I feel I am superwoman? Am I THAT amazing that resting because I have a headache over which I have no control such a failure?

I am alive, I want to be alive, I love life, living. I don't contemplate suicide, never really have. There were times I didn't want to live, sure, but I wanted to feel alive so there's that. This should be a good thing right? Wrong. Do I want a trophy for not wanting to kill myself? Most people do not want to kill themselves and they don't get a trophy. What is my point exactly?

I manage my home, (ish), my children are clean, fed, I have two cats, a stable marriage, I manage (very ish) to study my degree and/or work and when I do have a job I turn up, don't take sick days, I give it my all and I am usually quite darn good at it, people ask for my advice and in general like me. This is a good thing right? Wrong again. Keep up with the program will you? Most people do this anyway. This is how you *adult* and this is how you pay bills and raise your kids and aren't selling your body for cigarettes money stealing to maintain whatever habits people get into.

But wait… I do all those things even though I suffer from these things, I don't know, General Anxiety Disorder, Panic Attacks, Stress, Bipolar even. I don't get myself into unsurmountable debt when high and don't live in my bed and neglect my family when down. I do all these things and this should be good. Right? Again… Not quite. So what? Just because I am not weaker I should be happy with my mild weakness? O amy I am not strong at all. Maybe these people have it really bad and my forms of whatever I call "high functioning [insert disorder here] are just a sample and I will never know their true plight because I don't fully break down. Maybe I don't fully breakdown not because I am too strong but because I actually don't suffer as bad from this and am just finding excuses and crutches for my laziness and my meagreness and my unremarkableness and even my inability to deal.

3 MANIC? AND SAD? HOW?

Lately, well generally, I have been having these "mixed" feelings.

I used to her about *manic-depressive* and envisioned this. Exactly this. I am happy, manic even, hypo maybe, but still high. I am also desperate and sad and feel helpless and worthless and everything is kind of a failure, I am a failure. But also, isn't it a great day to be alive? I wanna do stuff, I wanna do stuff that will make me feel better and it will, it will all be ok because, because... well, because this song is amazing.

Chris Reinhardt

I was asked by a good friend today if I felt depressed. He's got a knack for these things. I wasn't. I managed to go to class yesterday and even though it was a stressful day, I was happy I went. I went and powered through and it was cool. It was ok. I was back and I was 'gonna catch up and all would be ok. But then I got up. And there was so much to do today, this week, this month, so many things I had no control over it and it would probably not be possible to do them all and it is all my fault… I told him I'd ring him later and speak to him for a bit but couldn't face it. Couldn't tell him how I felt like a failure and how when I answered his message, I wasn't depressed at all but now I was. For no reason whatsoever. He'd knew I was lying, and I'd have to try an explain why I was this way even though he get me and wouldn't ask. I'd have to try and hide how exactly shitty I felt, again, for no reason at all. So, I didn't call him. I'm certainly 'gonna make up some poorly thought and executed excuse about how busy I was or how I didn't have enough time for some reason I can't quite get into but, anyway, "how are you?"

4 I'M A MACHINE

I've just gotten home after spending all morning in my local café. I'm checking emails, logging in to accounts, solving things, on hold on a call I've been putting up for a few days now... I left the Robot Hoover on when I left in the morning so that's one last thing I must do. I also made sure my laptop was charging so I could do some work when returning. It's sunny outside and I'm stuck in here, but it's fine because I am being productive.

I love this side of my life. I love the "high functioning" description of it. I can get so much done. I can because I must in all honesty. I always have to but when I am down there is something missing, something which doesn't quite make its way into my brain, my body, my actions, something which says I can do it later, in a bit, tomorrow, next week, when I have time of patience. This seems wrong and stupid to me today as if I know it needs doing, I should just get on with it and do it, don't see a point in delaying it.

I am sure it won't last that long.

Maybe an hour, maybe a couple, maybe the whole day or maybe the whole week if the dead sleep time doesn't reset me into zombie mode. But it will stop. It will go away. And it makes me sad, it makes me annoyed, it makes me upset and even stressed.

Even writing this makes me stressed. I type quite quick, but today, quicker than most days as there is so much that needs going down on here and I fear it may leave me, the will to do it. The willingness. The ability.

As I was driving home, I was contemplating all the wonderful things I can do when I get home. There is some typing to do. The phone call I just finished which my amazing ability to put the questions and arguments got em a thorough and comprehensive explanation. Perhaps some actual lecture catch up and reading catch up, probably on immigration law which I find interesting but extremely bureaucratic and who know, maybe even a load or five of laundry before dinner. I feel accomplished with half a page and a phone call and am starting to have the distinct feeling I may not accomplish much more today.

I have, in the past, moved all my furniture around, made 3 different dinners which I packed and froze for emergencies, dyed my hair, did my back and/or front garden, cleared the clutter from cupboards, sorted all my desk and paperwork and shredded like Saul Godman's secretary towards the end of the series... I have been amazing. I can do this today. I don't need to move the furniture around and the work I have to do in the gardens requires my husbands help. I cleared my desk and the house clutter not that long and there is no need for it. I do need to dye my hair but haven't quite decided on the colour and am dead broke which always makes me self-conscious about spending money on stupid things like hair dye. Manicure. Waxing. New clothes or shoes for me. I have a feeling none of these things are ever necessary and I would be making myself a great disservice by getting them. I know I'd feel guilty. I still do it but feel shit after and have to go through a whole mental justification process. My husband doesn't really ask. He is ok with it. He's more on the normal side so understands that taking care of oneself by grooming and such of sorts isn't a bad thing. It's not gambling, it's not pissing my money away. Me... more of an acceptance proves is required still.

I'm not absolutely sure I want to get myself into the process of doing much. It may stress me and make me even more manic as is usually the case. I realise I'm amazing and test myself to see just how amazing. The feeling of accomplishment makes me happier and higher and I need to do something else after that. And something else after that. And something else after that. I can spend days, weeks in this. It's draining. The kids think I am mad, my husband love the sex but even he gets tired bless him, he loves the me being this productive but hates he can't sit till as I see it as a waste of life and the poor soul can't rest. It's great how my house looks in the end, how all my paperwork has been organized, emails answered, and phone calls returned. Uni work has been organized into sections and some actually done. The ones I've done I am doubtful about though, I am sure if I look at it later, *sober* I won't be as happy with the result but no one can have it all, it's done. The kids have their rooms in a proper and amazing state, maybe some redecorating took place, and mine looks relaxing, clean and a really nice place to sleep in. I have had time to see some of my friends and maybe we've been on a night out, I've been happy, chatty, hopeful.

I don't like what comes after. Sunshine before the storm is what this is. I fall long and hard. Sometimes I get physically unwell as my immune system that has been propelled on near pure adrenaline gives in and I get the cold and the cold sore. Other times I just get exhausted. Shattered. The chemicals are gone. I've used my allowance all at once and my brain decided to cut them off before I overdose. How my brain is kind and caring. I often mope around and don't have energy. No energy to cry most of the time. No patience. I just exist.

Chris Reinhardt

5 TODAY IS WEIRD

I am not the keenest on writing as I would write in a diary. I haven't held a diary since I was about 12. I've started them. I bought the notebooks, they were pretty or dark, or clever with reaffirming sentences on the cover but I just haven't seen benefits to it. I am very private about what goes on inside my brain and my heart and the fact that someone can read it and judge me is very present. I've done the electronic versions as well, started a couple of blogs, some I still write, some I lost interest, others I simply cannot come up with content I feel would match the tone of the blog....

Having said that, the more I write on here, the more I realise that because I want to make this as real as possible and edit as little as possible (only enough to make my ramblings intelligible) this is kind of what happens.

Today. Today I woke up happy. Slept well. Then events followed which would've floored me on a bad day, we are talking creditor issues… they rattled me but empowered me to go online and search *manically* for all these solutions I've been playing with in my brain. I feel crap. Life seems gloom. We are always broke, and this adds on so much to my issues, I couldn't even begin to say how much. However,… because I wasn't floored and had a proper meltdown, because I looked at solutions instead of dwelling on the problem I feel weird. It's probably because I am high on life still and see light at the end of the tunnel, but it's, well, WEIRD.

I feel despaired but energized to get out of my funk because I am wonder woman.

I feel sad because my life is in a chaos but feel it will get better because it has to and I rule.

I feel stressed and anxious, but quite clearheaded and my mental fog levels are very low. Maybe it's the adrenaline, maybe it's all the other chemicals I can barely pronounce but it is definitely something I have felt before and haven't been able to describe.

The uneducated ones in these matters – this is not a dig, I am uneducated in particle physics or how to build a house or make a perfect fold on a napkin to make into a swan and I don't feel dumb, I just don't know about that stuff – this must seem very abnormal. My rational brain part tells me I should be down and that it would be ok. When things go well, I should also feel well, and this would be ok. Feeling this mix of emotions is less easy to comprehend (yes, I know the word *harder* but the sentiment is different) and therefore, even though it is what I feel, harder (see) to accept. I can't even imagine how someone who has never felt anything like it, the *normal ones* are meant to understand it. How anyone is meant to accept that this is just a part of me, and I can't do much to change it. How I have learned to accept it the best I can and even, how given the chance, I am not sure I would change it because it's always been me.

Eminem said it best.

6 REALLY?! I'M NOT ALLOWED 'CAUSE YOU SAY SO?!

My Tom Cruise past obsession (s) – although can it be really called an obsession if it's only a few days long or if it goes unnoticed for years or you forget about it? – is about to be quenched. MI4 is on Prime. Now TV only had I, II and III which lasted me a couple of days, but 4, 4 with the beautiful Renner addition was missing from my *rewatch just because* list.

Well, tonight beaus, we gots a date.

Maybe this will make me happier. Simon Pegg has certainly already put a smile on my face, only about 3 min in. I needed it. I needed that smile. Today I posted on a Bipolar Support group online only to ask for material for an abstract video I was planning on making, with people's representations of their condition, maybe how messy or stupidly clean their house is, about how they feel or their tattoos… An abstract concept I haven't fully developed in my mind. Only to have said to me, by some self righteous person, how I could NOT – quite categorically – represent the Bip community. Why? Because she didn't agree with whatever synopsis she believed I had made of it. I didn't. Anyway, I am not justifying myself in writing for the second time today. My point: Because this one person doesn't agree with whatever they think I said, which was how people have misconceptions about it and I want to add to the discussion by shinning a light in the differences, I am now NOT ALLOWED to represent the community.

Who the f#ck does this b*tch think  she is?

I represent who the hell I want to represent. Just to be clear: Me! I represent me. If I resonate with someone else's feelings or experiences, brilliant. If people see in me a bit of them, or in them a bit of me, or if they read or see anything I write or do and think *sh*t, that's happened to me, I am not completely alone* then I am not a complete waste of space and all my life experiences weren't for nothing. I don't want to represent anyone or anything. I gave up that crap long ago. Basically, when I realized there are always at least three sides to every story and three versions of the truth in life. There is mine, yours and the real one. I can't represent yours and if mine and yours are different from the real one I can't represent that either. On a bad day, mine changes so even my representation of me isn't a completely faithful one.

Maybe only the might of Tom Cruise (don't argue, accept my truth and leave me be) can cure how I feel right now. The feeling of offence and indignation of this millennium is running through me at 10 min past midnight like caffeine and I really need to get some shut eye. Oh God how I hate feeling offended, attacked by self-righteous words… How it rattles me that it rattles me.

I have been through my fair share of online abuse, from people who *know* me, in their minds, and from people who live in my area, from people who – bless them – think they own the truth. It is a huge source of pride in me that over one year of this abuse received absolutely zero responses from me because I don't measure myself by the attitudes of others but by mine. Because I don't like lowering my level to the one of these people. Because I maybe think too highly of myself, but too highly or just the right amount of high, I do love myself in my own way and my competition is with me. My struggle, within. My enemy, myself. Others… I must share the whole planet with them, my life, I only have to share with a few and I get to choose those.

TODAY IS SH*T

I didn't get to choose my body, my family, the place I was born or raised in. Up to a certain age I wasn't really allowed to choose those who surrounded me and where I was being surrounded by them. I didn't get to choose my skin colour, my eye colour, my height, my body type, my health… my outer beauty or lack thereof. I didn't get to choose where I went to school, what I was taught or how I was taught. I don't get to choose which bills I pay, the size of the house I get to afford, the car I get to afford – barely get to choose one at all with what I can afford. But by the gods and the angels of all light and darkness, I get to f#cking chose whether to give the time of day to some people. I get to choose who gets my love, who gets my time, who gets me. Some people just don't. They don't get the real me. Some people don't get the fake me. Some people don't get any kind of me. Why I should dedicate a whole chapter to them is beyond me. So, in summary:

- Tom Cruise rules – I forgive him for his religious choices as they are his to make and don't affect me.
- Simon Pegg is great in the MI films and pretty much everything that isn't Paul – I don't judge so you shouldn't either.
- And Renner… Oh dear daddy, baby sweet face Renner… yes please.

7 IT SUCKS BEING A GIRL SOMETIMES

Hi boys. It's me. A girl. You guys have heard of menstruation and all the hormonal sh*t that comes with it. I am sure an overwhelming percentage of you have made PMS jokes, or in the least of leasts laughed at one. It's not a dig, calms down, I have. They're usually funny. Here's the thing though, when one of those b*tch days meets a b*tch mental health sh*t day… it's absolute Armageddon. Not some Walking Dead crap where Zombies move really slowly, not some World War Z where there is a cure, not the one where Bruce Willis saves the day or where Humanity can be saved… I am talking total destruction. Destruction of confidence, destruction of good mood or any mood which isn't bawling for no reason and every reason. Destruction of reasons to live, to clean the house, to go to class, to answer the phone, to get up, to wipe your eyes, to stop screaming inside – and often outside – destruction of any self-control when it comes to eating 3 chocolate filled doughnuts in a Lidl car park. And a lemon cheesecake lattice.

It took me most of the day to realise my period is due and that this wasn't the end of the world, I wasn't coming completely undone.

I am very tightly wound up and have been more so lately. This was not me falling through, not the cracks but, a giant whole in the earth. It was scary. It felt good for a bit. I got to cry. I don't do this much. I have found it very hard to let go – of everything really, but of crying – without it feeling like a flood. Today there was a flood. Today was one of those days.

I wanted to get my laptop out and write all these words in my head. Put all my worries on paper. Make a chapter about what was going on. I couldn't. I am glad I didn't. I am not even sure what it would look like. All the words raced through my head at such speed I am sure wouldn't be able to speak them so I wouldn't surely be able to type them. Even if I could, there were words on my head, much like now, but not so much sentences. Even now the delete key is starting to look at me funny as I struggle to make sentences about how I would struggle to make sentences.

I doubt I would want so much on paper

Chris Reinhardt

8 THIS IS NOT A GOOD CHAPTER

I believe, having written about 200 books in my mind and an absolute number of 0 (zero for clarification) on real life, that no one quite knows how their writing is going to end up. You have an idea. Things form in your head. I think different people will have different methods and it's possible some people have no method whatsoever. I am sure some people suffer from writers block and others cannot type fast enough. What I mean is that it must be a different experience for everyone, from self-help book writers to J.K and King.

I was toying with the idea of telling you a little bit about my process and how I feel alongside writing how I feel. Didn't feel productive. I also thought about, perhaps, telling you a little bit about my editing process, I did, a little bit already. And I was going to edit the least I could. I am now feeling I should really stop editing altogether. I did want, after all, this to be a realistic experiment of how my mental health affects me in various ways and my life in various ways. How it gives me the will to continue when most people would buckle and how painfully crippling it can be. I am writing in a particularly low and not to kind to myself period in my life though and have no wish for this to be a reflection of life in general. If my life in general.

I am saying I am not sure. I hope you don't hate me if I decide to leave my editing behind and if I don't go back and tidy chapters. There are now thoughts that haven't been finished for various reasons and chapters, much like this one which start nowhere and equally lead nowhere. I am not sure I am going to go back and *sort them out*.

Chris Reinhardt

9 MILLIONAIRE

It's not like I'd buy new friends like Monica suggested if she won the lottery, and wouldn't have the new ones have plastic surgery to look like the old ones but… I could invest and/or partner with most of them in some of their endeavors and they'd have more money, easier, freer lives. We could spend more time together and I could afford to call them up to my country house to play some tennis, squash or get drunk in a Thursday afternoon because they could. They didn't necessarily have to be in their shift or lose their job if they were hanging out with me. I could make sure they all had nice enough houses, there are a couple I'd buy them a little nice house or apartment for, and the other ones could just rent off me for a stupid low rent a really nice place. If our businesses did well, I wouldn't oppose on them having a "company car" and allowable expenses as part of their work benefits, lighten up their load a bit. Even paid holidays with the family once a year, why not? Happy workers are productive and loyal workers. How is this not money giving you some form of happiness?

I am sure I read somewhere that money does provide happiness regardless of what people think. I am talking serious research from some well-respected university. It makes sense to me. Not money that can buy you the biggest, most luxurious car, but money that buys you the car you like and that won't need the mechanic you can't afford every 3 months. Not the kind that will provide you with the mansion you can show off to your family, but the one where you have storage and your kids have privacy and your butler has their own walk in wardrobe, wait, what (?) - sorry got little distracted there – I mean one where you can have your friends over for an amazing BBQ which you can actually afford and where there is a guest place, bedroom, something where they can crash when they have too much to drink. Not the money that means you can send your kids to the best boarding or private schools but that where you don't have to worry about their school meal money for next week, or next months bus fare, or them growing out of their expensive uniforms or football boots. The one where you can send them to some private music lessons, or dance lessons, or no lessons, whatever, one where there is a choice.

So, I took a break after the last paragraph to… well, inevitably, look on Rightmove for amazing houses up to 5 mil 'cause, well, 'cause yes. Then I went to the loo and ended up not leaving for 20 min. Don't judge me, 5 min in the bathroom is too much for me, I am not one of those. I just needed a tinkle but spent the rest of the time designing my new bathroom in my mind for the millionth and second time, as you do. But guess what? I haven't any money. Also, days like today I haven't any motivation. I could have the money right now I would have no idea what to do with it. This is why I day dream a lot of a time when I'll be able to afford sh*t. It isn't all daydreaming of whatifs, it's mental prep people.

Stay with me here. We are told to save from the age of zero basically. We are taught to manage our money save for a rainy day, save for retirement, we have private pensions. We also have private health insurance (in the UK it's not really a thing, you don't really need it for your basic stuff), we have drivers' insurance, it is actually against the law to have any motor vehicle without insurance in a public road. We take out life insurance. WE insure our phones, our tv's and jewelry. Does this mean we wish for some bad thing to happen? No. We do this because of what if. And why? What are the chances? Well, the truth is that if there is one chance, there must be someone out there thinking, it won't be them, and BAM, some day it is.

TODAY IS SH*T

We are not taught ho to prepare for good things. We are not taught what to do if we get a really nice job with quite a nice wage, how to plan, invest, manage. We are not taught what to do f we get an inheritance from a rich uncle we didn't know we had. If we marry a rich partner, which is why so many relationships where there is disparity in class, money go down the crap, because people are not prepared. Same with winning any kind of lottery. If we get a really nice tidy sum that gets outs a clean slate, a paid for generous house, a nice car and some really nice holidays with a new wardrobe to match we might be ok. Or just the holiday money. But… What about the ridiculous amounts of money people get? How do you deal with that? How do you decide if you move town or country or stay where you are? How do you know if you want a classic house or a new modern build when money is virtually no objection? Cars? How do you decide on that when the most expensive thing you had was about a couple months wage paid for in instalments? I am pretty sure it must be really hard to deal. And this my lovely people, therefore I plan. I plan about everything, so why shouldn't I plan for this? I have a basic idea of what house we'd buy for a family home, we'd build in our home country, we'd buy a couple of city places in London and back home of course, in the beach, in the capital. Maybe one or two little holiday places in a couple of European cities although not right way, we'd have to visit the place and fall in love. These are longer term plans. We need land and character so something in a village and not a new build preferably, although I saw one last year I'd buy in a blink. We'd definitely stop for two ticks and make the quickest of plans depending on the amount – we'd round it up and get a couple of millions available with no compromises, buy a stupidly expensive dress, piece of useless jewelry, a vase, don't care. This would be "unaccounted" money that would not be part of the plan and we could go crazy with it, get it our of our systems. We'd instantly put some on trust for the children, sizeable amounts which they could only get at 18, 21, 25, 20, after getting married, only to use in studies, or a house, or in their wedding… I am very specific, I wouldn't want them squandering it all away and end up struggling in the future. I'd get some aside for us in bonds or whatever (enlist banker and accountant here) for our retirement. We'd decide on a max for the house and the houses in general. We'd set how much we'd want to give our parents and extended family and friends. We'd decide how much we think we'd need for utilities and food and etc. and make sure we'd need that amount every month for however many years. After all this, couple of weeks I think, we'd go on a stupidly expensive holiday somewhere followed by a relaxing non timed holiday back home, depending on kids schooling we'd have to move back and forth but you get the point. We'd not invest, buy stupid things, only buy the cars we need – I want two (probably a Range Rover Autobiography Supercharged V8 in pure black and a Jaguar XF, maybe SW, not too bothered and hubby can have a normal one whichever one hen… TIRED. I am TIRED already. Therefore I need to plan when I am not depressed or hyper…

Moving on.

TODAY IS SH*T

10 THE END... OF THIS WEEK

This has indeed been an interesting 8 days. I wasn't sure how long I was going to be able to keep this up for or if I'd finish. I have. I didn't decide on a week to start with. I didn't decide on much to start with. I wanted to write a non-journal, a non-8-year-old-diary type something that I could share with people. Something which was real. But I didn't want to share much. I share so much but I share nothing. There are about 2 people that know me in this entire world and even to them I don't talk as much as I should. I feel safe around a fair amount of people, but I can't share certain aspect of certain things with them. I have different friends for different moods, I have different people in my life for my different me(s). I don't use them, not anymore than any of use use others, nor do I seek them out specifically, but they all 'gotta fir somewhere. If they don't, they're not really in my life.

I wanted to write something which would give an insight into how difficult it is sometimes for others to keep their sh*t together. We don't all fall apart all the time but we most definitely don't all have it all together all the time. I am guilty of wishing for peace of mind, for stability and often wishing it because it seems apparent in others and I want that. I am sure these *others* often wish my own apparent happiness, stability, strength, certainly in just being. I hope these strings of letters which sometimes resemble words and more often than not don't even remotely resemble sentences, can help you. I hope you related a little bit. I hope I made some sense at some point. IF you didn't relate, I hope you understood there are people out there like me, who are too afraid to speak up, who are too afraid of letting go, even just for a second, who are falling apart inside just waiting to be found out as the frauds they feel. I hope you are kinder to people because you never know who they may be.

Depression, Bipolar, Mood and Panic disorders, Agoraphobias, other phobias, all phobias, Stress, Anxiety and Stress and Anxiety... All the others I am not going to enumerate or make up acronyms for, all those things exist, they are out there in people. IN people. Inside them. And everyday you meet an Uber driver, a checkout person, a Dr or a nurse, a teacher, a Starbucks attendant or a cleaning lady to whom these issues are real. Everyday you walk past a house where someone is crying inside, sunk in their disgusting bed they haven't changed the sheets of for months in a deep state of depression and even contemplating suicide. Everyday you will see someone who has just wiped the tears of their face so strangers wouldn't see them. Everyday you see someone with greasy unwashed hair or overdone make up because they were too sad to shower or wanted to make sure people thought they had it all figured out and wore that perfectly overdone makeup as a war mask. Everyday you see these people and they see you. Maybe you are the one I am referring to. The shadow of mental health casts no real shadow and can't therefore be seen.

You can help someone elderly crossing the street because you see they are struggling at life, you can donate to someone homeless or buy them a hot drink because you see their plight. You can do a fun run for someone who lost a limb and needs a prosthetic one. You can donate money on your phone to abandoned animals or children in need.

You cannot do this for any ONE person with mental health. You don't know who they are. What is wrong with them. You cannot give them a hand because the road they need to cross is not literal. You cannot buy us a comforting hot anything because the comfort we require is often ethereal and not physical, you probably wouldn't know we need a comforting anything as we wouldn't tell you and you can't just guess. You can't do a fun run for us, it won't get us maid to do the housework we can't bear to do, or pay our bills because we are too ill to work, it is not seen as a struggle most of the time and most people still believe we need to just "nap out of it". You can't really donate anything to

TODAY IS SH*T

us as we don't tell you we need it, would be too proud to accept it or accept it and feel even sh*ttier after. The donations we need are things which the world doesn't have much of. We nee love. We need understanding. We need time. These are things that can't be bought, things that can't be donated, loaned, and therefore they are so hard to get. They require actual human investment. I hope you find it in you to invest in people around you, who knows if one of them is in real need.

Even if you are one of the ones in need, still make an effort. Sometimes we need others and sometimes other need us just a little bit more. Being needed is also therapy.

I hope you can forgive me for my rants and very little or in places, total lack of edit and consistency but reality is neither.

B good, B well, B happy.

Chris Reinhardt

ABOUT THE AUTHOR

    I speak quite a lot. I also tell a lot of stories and retell them to the non-amusement of most of the people around me. I tend to overshare. I do this on facts. Most people, therefore, feel they know me pretty well. They don't. I seldom share feelings. I pondered how much to insert in here and decided pretty much against EVERYTHING. I still fear… something. I fear the ignorance and unwillingness of people and their reactions to things they don't know, understand or have no wish to do so. Whatever demons I have in me, I'm keeping them my own for now.

    If you feel this is something you struggle with as well, if you overcame this, if you agree or disagree, or if you are just bored, drop me a line at my very cleaver named non-descriptive email below.

    Todayissh8t@hotmail.com

www.ingramcontent.com/pod-product-compliance
Lightning Source LLC
Chambersburg PA
CBHW081024170526
45158CB00010B/3144